VIAGRA MED

The essential guide to l(

everything about Viagra ... wonder

blue pill for treating erectile

dysfunction, improve sex drive and

enjoy long lasting sex

Dr Billy Rich

Table of contents

CHAPTER ONE

Introduction

Innumerable facets of human health have been revolutionized as a result of the remarkable advances in modern medicine. Viagra is a beacon of optimism and transformation in the realms of sexual health and relationships among these revolutionary advances. Initially discovered as a potential treatment for a different medical condition, this emblematic blue drug has become a symbol of revitalized intimacy and vitality for individuals and couples.

Viagra has emerged as a catalyst for bringing down barriers and promoting frank dialogues about sexual health in a culture that is often reluctant to discuss such matters. Its voyage from laboratory discovery to ubiquitous name exemplifies not only scientific ingenuity, but also the fundamental significance of maintaining healthy relationships and embracing holistic well-being.

In this investigation, we delve into the complex science underlying Viagra's mechanism of action, casting light on how it targets the physiological factors that contribute to erectile dysfunction. Beyond its physiological effects, we will explore the profound impact that Viagra has on the emotional and psychological dimensions of relationships by examining the experiences of couples who have personally witnessed its transformative effects.

As we progress through the pages of this investigation, we will also address important considerations, such as the safety of Viagra use, the possibility of adverse effects, and the significance of consulting with medical professionals. In addition, we will examine Viagra's role as a forerunner of innovative solutions and its potential contributions to the ongoing evolution of sexual health.

Join us as we uncover the intricate connections between scientific innovation, emotional rejuvenation, and the intricate web of human relationships. We will examine, through the lens of Viagra, how this remarkable drug has not only reshaped the landscape of sexual health but also inspired dialogues that promote understanding, empathy, and a renewed sense of connection.

Brief history of Viagra's discovery and development

Viagra, also known as sildenafil citrate, was discovered and developed at a captivating intersection of medical research and unanticipated outcomes. Here is a concise summary of its history:

Originating as a Cardiovascular Drug: Pfizer conducted research on a class of compounds known as PDE5 inhibitors during the late 1980s. Initially, these compounds were investigated for their potential to treat cardiovascular conditions such as angina and hypertension. Viagra's active constituent, sildenafil, was one of these compounds.

During clinical trials of sildenafil as a potential cardiovascular medication, researchers observed an unanticipated adverse effect: an increase in penile erections among male participants. Although the compound did not demonstrate significant efficacy for its intended cardiovascular purpose, it had a significant effect on erectile function.

Recognizing the potential significance of this side effect, Pfizer shifted its attention from cardiovascular applications to the treatment of erectile dysfunction (ED), a condition affecting millions of men. In 1998, the U.S. Food and Drug Administration (FDA) authorized Pfizer to market sildenafil under the brand name Viagra as the first oral treatment for erectile dysfunction (ED).

4. Commercial Success and Cultural Impact

The 1998 introduction of Viagra was a watershed moment in the field of sexual health. Its introduction brought ED to the forefront of public discourse, thereby reducing stigma and encouraging discussions about sexual health. The capsule in the shape of a blue diamond acquired widespread recognition and became a cultural phenomenon very rapidly.

Following the triumph of Viagra, other pharmaceutical companies developed their own PDE5 inhibitors for the treatment of erectile dysfunction. In addition, ongoing research investigated the potential benefits of sildenafil for other conditions, including pulmonary arterial hypertension (PAH), a form of elevated blood pressure affecting the arteries of the lungs.

6. Generic Versions and Global Availability: In the years following the expiration of Pfizer's patent for sildenafil, generic versions of Viagra became available, making treatment for erectile dysfunction (ED) more accessible to individuals. The availability of generics has helped make medication more affordable and accessible in various regions of the globe.

Beyond its well-known use for erectile dysfunction, sildenafil has been investigated for its potential therapeutic effects in a variety of medical conditions, including Raynaud's phenomenon, altitude sickness, and even some forms of cancer. The investigation of these possible applications continues.

The discovery and development of Viagra illustrate the unpredictability of scientific research and the potential for unanticipated results to lead to revolutionary advancements. What began as an investigation into cardiovascular health paved the way for a medication that has not only enhanced the lives of innumerable individuals and couples, but also spurred discussions about sexual health and relationships more broadly.

CHAPTER TWO

Importance of addressing sexual health in relationships

It is essential to address sexual health in relationships in order to cultivate emotional intimacy, maintain overall well-being, and promote a healthy partnership. Here are some of the most important reasons why managing sexual health is of the uttermost importance:

Sexual intimacy is a fundamental aspect of romantic relationships, as it enables partners to express their love, vulnerability, and affection. Open communication about sexual desires, needs, and concerns facilitates the development of a stronger emotional bond between partners, leading to greater trust and mutual understanding.

Sexual satisfaction has a close relationship with overall relationship fulfillment. When both partners feel satisfied and connected in their erotic experiences, it frequently translates to greater happiness and contentment in other areas of the relationship.

Promoting effective communication is essential for discussing sexual health. Engaging in these discussions encourages partners to become more at ease with discussing sensitive topics, establishing a positive precedent for confronting other crucial issues within the relationship.

Regular conversations about sexual health enable couples to identify and address any potential concerns or obstacles as early as possible. Couples can work toward resolving issues and prevent them from escalating if they acknowledge and confront problems together.

5. Navigating Life Transitions: Throughout life, various factors can affect sexual health, including physical health changes, hormonal shifts, stress, and changes in lifestyle. Openly discussing these changes allows couples to adapt and discover new methods to maintain intimacy and connection.

6. Contributing to Total Well-Being A thriving sexual existence can support total well-being. Regular sexual activity has been associated with physical

benefits such as reduced tension, enhanced immune function, and improved cardiovascular health. In addition, the release of oxytocin during intimate interactions fosters feelings of closeness and relaxation.

7. Challenging Stigma and Misconceptions: Open dialogues about sexual health assist in challenging societal stigmas and misconceptions regarding topics such as erectile dysfunction, low libido, and sexual preferences. This can contribute to a relationship environment that is more tolerant and inclusive.

Addressing sexual health concerns in the context of a supportive relationship can enhance an individual's self-esteem and confidence. Partners who collaborate actively to surmount obstacles can develop a greater sense of self-worth.

Unresolved sexual issues can cause resentment, frustration, and misunderstandings between partners. Open communication regarding sexual needs and desires prevents these destructive emotions from accumulating and harming the relationship.

Promoting Relationship Satisfaction Over time, both relationships and sexual dynamics change. Addressing sexual health throughout a relationship ensures that both partners feel valued and prioritized, which contributes to the relationship's long-term satisfaction and longevity.

In essence, addressing sexual health involves creating a secure and supportive environment in which partners can communicate openly, express their desires and concerns, and collaborate to ensure mutual satisfaction. Couples can cultivate a strong and resilient alliance that endures the measure of time by recognizing the significance of sexual health within the context of a relationship.

CHAPTER THREE

How Viagra works to enhance erectile function

Viagra (sildenafil citrate) is a revolutionary drug that has improved the lives of innumerable men with erectile dysfunction (ED), which is the inability to obtain or maintain an erection sufficient for satisfactory sexual performance. Viagra has given individuals and couples a new lease on life through its targeted mechanism of action, restoring intimacy, bolstering self-confidence, and rekindling emotional connections. To comprehend how Viagra works, one must delve into the complex interaction between physiology, biochemistry, and pharmacology.

The Route to Erection: An Intricate Symphony

Achieving and maintaining an erection is a complex physiological process that requires the coordination of multiple systems. The circulatory system, specifically the complex network of blood vessels in the penis, is central to this process. The relaxation of smooth muscles within the penis and the consequent increase in blood flow to the erectile tissues are necessary for a successful erection.

Nitric Oxide: The Primary Ignitor

The path to a robust and long-lasting erection begins with sexual arousal, which is activated by sensory or mental stimulation. In response, nerve signals travel from the brain to the genital region, triggering the release of nitric oxide (NO) from the endothelial cells surrounding the blood vessels in the penis.

Nitric oxide is essential for vasodilation, the expansion and relaxation of blood vessels. This improves circulation to the erectile tissues by allowing more blood to circulate through them. The release of NO initiates a chain of biochemical reactions that result in the relaxation of smooth muscle cells in the penile artery and cavernous body walls.

The Function of Phosphodiesterase Type 5

While nitric oxide initiates the vasodilation process, phosphodiesterase type 5 (PDE5) serves as a natural counterbalance.

PDE5 is an enzyme that degrades cyclic guanosine monophosphate (cGMP), the molecule responsible for smooth muscle cell relaxation. As cGMP levels fall as a result of PDE5 activity, smooth muscles in the penis constrict, impeding blood flow and causing the erection to subside.

Viagra's Action Mechanism: A Molecular Intervention

This is where Viagra enters the picture. Viagra's active constituent, sildenafil citrate, is classified as a PDE5 inhibitor. It interferes with the normal function of the PDE5 enzyme due to its presence in the body. Viagra inhibits the rapid degradation of cGMP by inhibiting PDE5, allowing cGMP levels to remain elevated for a prolonged time.

As cGMP levels continue to rise, the smooth muscles in the penile blood vessels remain calm, resulting in an increase in blood flow to the erectile tissues. The outcome is a sustained, robust, and long-lasting erection.

The Importance of Timing and Precision in Sexual Stimulation

Noting that Viagra's effectiveness depends on sexual arousal is essential. The medication does not induce spontaneous erections; rather, it enhances the natural response of the body to sexual stimulation. Sexual arousal activates the cGMP pathway by causing the release of nitric oxide. Viagra enhances this process by sustaining elevated levels of cGMP, thereby prolonging and intensifying the response to sexual stimuli.

Dosage, Timing, and Factors to Consider

Viagra is typically available in quantities spanning from 25 to 100 milligrams. Individual factors such as age, overall health, and the severity of erectile dysfunction determine the appropriate dosage. It is essential to adhere to the dosage and directions provided by a healthcare professional.

Viagra is typically administered orally 30 to 60 minutes prior to sexual activity. The onset of action varies from individual to individual, and factors such as a high-fat meal may delay the medication's efficacy. To ensure optimal results, it is recommended to avoid hefty meals and extensive alcohol consumption before taking Viagra.

Safety and Possible Adverse Effects

Similar to other medications, Viagra may cause certain adverse effects. Headache, facial flushing, nasal congestion, gastritis, and mild visual disturbances are typical side effects. In general, these adverse effects are moderate and transient. Rarely, however, more severe side effects such as sudden vision or hearing loss, protracted erections (priapism), and cardiovascular problems may occur. If you experience unusual or severe symptoms, you must seek medical attention immediately.

A Portal to Intimacy and Self-Assurance

The action mechanism of Viagra is a triumph of scientific knowledge and innovation. By selectively inhibiting PDE5, Viagra enables men with erectile dysfunction to attain and maintain gratifying erections through a natural and regulated process. Viagra has had a profound impact on relationships, self-esteem, and overall well-being, in addition to its physiological effects.

Viagra has been a lifeline for individuals and couples affected by erectile dysfunction, opening doors to intimacy, communication, and a renewed sense of connection. As our understanding of sexual health evolves, Viagra remains a compelling example of the potential for medical advances to transform lives, redefine relationships, and restore the pleasure of physical and emotional intimacy.

Prevalence of Erectile Dysfunction (ED)

Erectile dysfunction (ED) is a prevalent medical condition that impacts a substantial proportion of men worldwide. It is the consistent inability to attain or maintain an erection adequate for satisfying sexual performance. The prevalence of erectile dysfunction increases with age, but this is not solely due to aging. Physical, psychological, and lifestyle factors, among others, contribute to its occurrence.

The prevalence of erectile dysfunction can vary based on various studies and populations, but it is estimated that: • Approximately 40% of men at age 40 experience some degree of erectile dysfunction; • The prevalence increases to approximately 70% in men aged 70 and older.

These statistics emphasize the significant impact of erectile dysfunction on the male population and the need for effective interventions and treatments.

Impact of Eating Disorders on Relationships

ED can have profound emotional, psychological, and relational consequences beyond its physiological effects. It affects not only the individual experiencing the condition, but also their companions and the relationship's overall dynamics. Listed below are some ways that ED can impact relationships:

ED can result in frustration, humiliation, and a feeling of inadequacy. These emotions may impede open communication between partners regarding their sexual health and desires, resulting in emotional distance and a decrease in intimacy.

Sexual intimacy is a fundamental component of romantic relationships. When ED hinders the ability to engage in sexual activity, couples may experience a decline in physical intimacy, resulting in feelings of disconnection and a strain on their emotional attachment.

Loss of Confidence and Self-Esteem: Men with erectile dysfunction may experience a significant loss of confidence and self-esteem. This can impact their sense of masculinity and contribute to feelings of insignificance, which may manifest in other areas of their existence.

ED can contribute to psychological problems such as anxiety, depression, and performance anxiety. These conditions can exacerbate the difficulties of ED and have an effect on both the individual and the relationship.

5. Relationship Tension and Resentment Unresolved ED-related issues can lead to relationship tension, conflicts, and even resentment. Unmet expectations and discontent can burden the relationship, generating a cycle of tension and conflict.

Partners of individuals with an eating disorder may internalize the situation and doubt their own desirability or attractiveness. They may erroneously attribute the condition to a lack of interest in them, adding to their emotional distress.

Sexual Dissatisfaction: Erectile dysfunction can result in sexual experiences that are unsatisfying for both partners. This can result in a decline in sexual gratification, which may have an effect on the overall satisfaction of the relationship.

8. Obstacles to Seeking Help Stigma and misconceptions about eating disorders may prevent people from seeking help or discussing the issue openly. This reluctance to confront the

issue can perpetuate the relationship's negative effects.

Seeking Support and Solutions

To address the impact of ED on relationships, frank communication, empathy, and a willingness to work together to find solutions are required. Seeking professional assistance from healthcare providers, therapists, or counselors can provide valuable guidance and techniques for coping with the emotional and relational aspects of ED.

In recent years, Viagra (sildenafil) has provided effective options for treating erectile dysfunction and restoring sexual function. Medication such as Viagra can assist men in regaining their confidence, enhancing their ability to engage in sexual activity, and ultimately improving relationship dynamics.

By recognizing the multifaceted impact of ED on relationships and taking proactive measures to address the physical, emotional, and relational dimensions, couples can successfully navigate this challenge together, nurturing understanding, intimacy, and a renewed sense of connection.

CHAPTER FOUR

Viagra Dosage

Viagra (sildenafil citrate) is available in a variety of concentrations, each designed to accommodate varying degrees of erectile dysfunction (ED) severity and specific patient requirements. The appropriate dosage of Viagra depends on variables such as the patient's age, general health, response to the medication, and potential drug interactions. Viagra should only be taken under the supervision and with a prescription from a qualified healthcare professional. Here are the most common Viagra dosages:

1. 25 mg: This is the lowest permissible dosage. Individuals who are sensitive

to the effects of sildenafil or who are taking medications that may interact with higher doses frequently receive this medication. Also appropriate for individuals with moderate erectile dysfunction.

50 mg is the standard starting dose and is effective for the majority of men with mild to moderate erectile dysfunction. This dosage is frequently the starting point for treatment, and it may be adjusted based on the individual's response.

100 milligrams is the maximum dosage available for Viagra. Typically prescribed to men with more severe erectile dysfunction or those who have not achieved adequate results with reduced doses.

It is essential to adhere to your healthcare provider's dosing instructions. Viagra is typically administered 30 minutes to 1 hour prior to sexual activity. For optimal results, it is recommended to take Viagra on an empty stomach, as high-fat meals can delay the medication's effects.

Keep in mind that Viagra should only be consumed once per day. Before modifying the dosage or frequency of use, it is vital to consult with your healthcare provider if the prescribed dosage is not producing the intended results or if you experience adverse effects.

• Age: Due to potential differences in metabolism and general health, elderly patients may require different dosages.

• Medical History: When determining the appropriate dosage, your healthcare provider will consider any underlying medical conditions, medications you are taking, and potential drug interactions.

• Response to Treatment: After attempting a particular dosage, your healthcare provider may alter it based on your response and any adverse effects you experience.

Prior to beginning or modifying any medication, including Viagra, it is crucial to prioritize safety and consult a healthcare professional. They will evaluate your unique situation and provide individualized advice to ensure that you receive the most effective and secure treatment for your erectile dysfunction.

potiential side effects on Viagra

Viagra (sildenafil citrate) is generally safe and effective in the treatment of erectile dysfunction (ED). Similar to other medications, it may cause adverse effects spanning from mild to rare and severe. Before using Viagra, it is necessary to be aware of these potential adverse effects and to consult a healthcare professional. Here are a few of the potential adverse effects of Viagra:

Frequent Adverse Effects: These adverse effects are relatively common, typically moderate, and transient. They may consist of:

Headache is a common adverse effect that is frequently caused by the medication's increased blood flow.

Some people may experience facial flushing, which is a sensation of warmth and discoloration of the epidermis on the face.

Viagra can induce nasal congestion or nasal discharge in some individuals.

Indigestion or Upset Stomach: Gastrointestinal discomfort, such as indigestion, reflux, or upset stomach, is possible.

Some individuals may experience moderate vertigo or a sensation of lightheadedness.

Less Frequent Adverse Effects: These adverse effects are less frequent but still possible:

Vision Alterations Viagra may cause vision alterations, such as impaired vision, sensitivity to light, or altered color perception. Rarely, more severe vision problems have been reported.

Back Pain or Muscle Aches: Some people may experience back pain or muscle aches, which are typically mild and temporary.

Rare and Severe Adverse Effects: Although uncommon, these adverse effects can be severe and require prompt medical attention:

Priapism is a protracted and occasionally excruciating erection that lasts longer than four hours. Priapism necessitates immediate medical attention to forestall possible penile injury.

Sudden Vision or Hearing Loss: A sudden decline or loss of vision or hearing that may indicate a serious medical condition. Consult a physician if this occurs.

In uncommon instances, Viagra may result in alterations in blood pressure or cardiac rate. Seek immediate medical attention if you experience chest pain, shortness of breath, or any other symptoms of a heart condition.

4. Allergic Reactions: Although extremely uncommon, some people may experience allergic reactions to Viagra, including rash, irritation,

puffiness, severe vertigo, and difficulty breathing.

This list is not exhaustive, and individual responses to Viagra may vary. If you experience any severe or unusual adverse effects while taking Viagra, you should immediately discontinue use and seek medical attention.

Prior to taking Viagra or any other medication for erectile dysfunction, it is essential to have a thorough discussion with a healthcare professional. They can evaluate your medical history, current medications, and overall health to determine whether or not Viagra is safe and suitable for you. If prescribed, they will provide instructions on proper use, potential adverse effects, and any precautions that are necessary.

Importance of consulting healthcare professionals before use

Prior to using any medication, including Viagra (sildenafil citrate), it is crucial to consult a healthcare professional for multiple reasons.

Healthcare professionals can conduct a thorough evaluation of your medical history, current health status, and any existing medical conditions. This evaluation helps determine whether Viagra is an appropriate and safe option for you, taking into account potential drug interactions and underlying health conditions.

2. Appropriate Dosage and Administration: Health care professionals can recommend the correct dosage of Viagra based on your individual requirements and response. It is essential to take the correct dosage to achieve the desired results while minimizing the risk of adverse effects.

Certain medical conditions, such as cardiovascular disease, high blood pressure, or a history of certain ocular disorders, may render the use of Viagra dangerous or contraindicated. A healthcare provider can identify these hazards and recommend safer alternatives or treatments.

4.Management of Side EffectsHealthcare professionals can

provide you with information on Viagra's potential side effects and how to manage them. They can advise you on whether particular adverse effects are normal, when you should seek medical attention, and how to alleviate discomfort.

Viagra can interact with other medications, potentially causing adverse effects or reducing the efficacy of either drug. Your current medication regimen can be reviewed by a healthcare professional to identify and manage potential drug interactions.

Occasionally, erectile dysfunction is a symptom of an underlying health condition, such as diabetes, hormonal imbalances, or cardiovascular disease. A healthcare provider can assist in identifying and treating these root causes, thereby enhancing your overall health and wellbeing.

If you have a history of allergies or sensitivities to certain medications, a healthcare professional can determine if Viagra is safe for you and whether you need to take any precautions.

Individualized advice: each person's health status is unique. A healthcare provider can provide individualized guidance and treatment recommendations based on your unique health circumstances, allowing you to make informed treatment decisions.

Regular check-ups and follow-up appointments with healthcare professionals allow them to monitor your progress, modify the treatment plan as needed, and address any concerns or questions you may have.

Safe and Effective Treatment: Receiving erectile dysfunction treatment under the supervision of a healthcare professional ensures that you will receive a safe and effective treatment. They can provide evidence-based recommendations and assist you in making choices that are in line with your health objectives.

In conclusion, for your safety, well-being, and optimal treatment outcomes, you must consult a healthcare professional prior to taking Viagra or any other medication. Expertise, personalized assessment, and direction from a healthcare provider contribute to a holistic approach to managing your health and addressing any issues related to erectile dysfunction.

CHAPTER FIVE

Medical consultation and prescription requirements

Before using medications such as Viagra (sildenafil citrate), a consultation with a physician and a prescription are essential. These requirements are intended to guarantee patient safety, proper medication use, and optimal treatment outcomes. Here is a summary of the Viagra consultation and prescription procedure:

• Before beginning any treatment for erectile dysfunction, it is essential to have an in-person consultation with a qualified healthcare professional. This could be a primary care physician, urologist, or men's health specialist.The healthcare provider will inquire about your medical history, current medications, lifestyle practices, and any existing health conditions during the consultation. This exhaustive analysis assists in identifying potential hazards and contraindications.

Physical Examination:The healthcare professional may evaluate blood pressure, pulse rate, and other pertinent health indicators.

3. Discussion of Symptoms: • Patients should discuss openly their erectile dysfunction-related symptoms, including the frequency and severity of the problem, any emotional or psychological impact, and any other pertinent concerns.

4. Underlying Health Conditions: • The healthcare provider will screen for any

underlying health conditions that may be contributing to erectile dysfunction, such as diabetes, cardiovascular disease, hormonal imbalances, or neurological problems.

• It is essential to provide a comprehensive inventory of all medications, including over-the-counter medicines, supplements, and herbal remedies. Viagra may interact with certain medications, resulting in adverse effects.

6. Allergies and Sensitivities: • Inform the healthcare provider of any medication or substance allergies or sensitivities.

7. Education and Information: • The healthcare professional will provide information about Viagra, including its

mechanism of action, proper usage, potential adverse effects, and precautions for using the medication.

8.Issuance of a Prescription: If the healthcare provider determines that Viagra is safe and appropriate for your circumstance, they will issue a prescription with the recommended dosage and usage instructions.

Follow-Up and Monitoring: • Following the initiation of Viagra treatment, you may be scheduled for regular follow-up appointments to monitor your response, examine any adverse effects, and make any necessary adjustments to the treatment plan.

It is essential to follow the dosage and administration instructions supplied by the healthcare provider. Never take

Viagra or any other medication without a prescription from a licensed physician.

Viagra's consultation and prescription requirements are in place to prioritize patient safety and ensure that the medication is used in accordance with individual health requirements. By adhering to these guidelines, patients can benefit from a more individualized and effective approach to treating erectile dysfunction, while minimizing potential risks and complications.

Managing side effects

Although many individuals tolerate Viagra (sildenafil citrate) well, it is still essential to be aware of the possibility of adverse reactions. If you experience any of these side effects, it is advised that you consult a healthcare professional. Here are some potential Viagra adverse effects and management strategies:

• Headaches are a common adverse effect of Viagra, frequently resulting from increased blood flow.

• Managing: OTC pain relievers may help relieve moderate headaches. Assuring adequate hydration and slumber can also be beneficial.

• Some people may experience facial flushing, which is characterized by a warm, crimson sensation in the face and neck.

• Management: Typically, flushing is transitory and innocuous. Keeping calm, staying hydrated, and avoiding triggers such as alcohol and heated beverages may be beneficial.

Congestion of the Nasal Passages: •
Viagra can produce nasal congestion or
a congested nose.

• Treatment: OTC decongestants and
saline nasal mists may provide relief.
Additionally, staying hydrated can help
clarify mucus and alleviate congestion.

Indigestion or unsettled Stomach: •
Gastrointestinal discomfort, such as
indigestion or unsettled stomach, is a
possibility.

• Managing: Taking Viagra with a
modest meal or on an empty stomach
may decrease the likelihood of gastritis.
Also helpful is avoiding fattening or
piquant foods before taking the
medication.

5. Vertigo or Lightheadedness: • Some people may experience moderate vertigo or lightheadedness.

• Managing: To reduce the risk of vertigo, avoid sudden changes in position (such as rising up rapidly). If symptoms persist or worsen, you should consult a doctor.

Vision Changes: • Viagra may cause temporary vision changes, such as impaired vision, light sensitivity, or altered color perception.

• Managing: If you experience vision changes, do not engage in activities requiring clear vision until the symptoms subside. Consult a doctor if vision changes are severe or persistent.

Back Pain or Muscle Soreness: • Some people may experience moderate back pain or muscle soreness.

• Managing: OTC pain relievers, rest, and moderate stretching exercises can alleviate pain.

• Priapism is a rare but severe side effect characterized by an agonizing erection that lasts longer than four hours.

• Managing: Seek immediate medical attention if you experience priapism, as delayed treatment can result in irreversible damage.

• Although extremely uncommon, sudden vision or hearing loss has been reported as a possible side effect.

• Managing: If you experience sudden vision or hearing loss, you should immediately stop taking Viagra and seek medical assistance.

10. Allergic Reactions: Allergic reactions to Viagra are uncommon, but can include rash, irritation, puffiness, severe vertigo, and respiratory difficulties.

• Management: If you experience any symptoms of an allergic reaction, discontinue use of Viagra and seek immediate medical attention.

It is essential to keep in mind that not everyone will experience these adverse effects, and that many individuals tolerate Viagra without significant problems. However, if you do experience any adverse effects, you should seek advice from your healthcare provider. In addition, never alter the dosage or frequency of Viagra without first consulting your healthcare provider. They are able to provide individualized recommendations for managing adverse effects and ensuring a safe and effective treatment experience.

CHAPTER FIVE

Interactions with other medications and substances

Viagra (sildenafil citrate) interactions with other medications or substances can potentially affect the medication's efficacy and safety. Before commencing Viagra, it is crucial to inform your healthcare provider of all medications, supplements, and substances you are taking. Here are some interactions to keep in mind:

• Combining Viagra with nitrates, which are commonly used to treat chest pain (angina), can cause a hazardous decline in blood pressure. This combination can result in hypotension, a potentially fatal condition.Never use Viagra if you are taking nitroglycerin in any form (tablets, patches, aerosols, or ointments).

Alpha Blockers: • Alpha-blocker medications, which are frequently used to treat excessive blood pressure or prostate enlargement, can interact with Viagra and cause a significant decrease in blood pressure.

• Combining alpha-blockers and Viagra requires medical supervision and dosage modification.

• Combining Viagra with other erectile dysfunction medications, such as Cialis (tadalafil) or Levitra (vardenafil), can increase the risk of adverse effects and complications.

4. Protease Inhibitors (HIV Medications): • Protease inhibitors used to treat HIV can increase the levels of

Viagra in the circulation, which may increase the risk of adverse effects.

• Certain medications used to treat fungal infections (ketoconazole, itraconazole) or bacterial infections (erythromycin) can impact the way Viagra is metabolized, resulting in increased blood levels of the drug.

6. Grapefruit and Grapefruit Juice: • Grapefruit and grapefruit juice can inhibit the enzyme responsible for metabolizing Viagra, resulting in elevated blood concentrations of the medication. This may increase the likelihood of adverse effects.

Alcohol: • Consuming alcoholic beverages while taking Viagra can increase the risk of certain adverse effects, especially vertigo and low blood pressure.

• The use of recreational drugs, especially substances that affect blood pressure or cardiovascular function, can interact with Viagra and pose significant health risks.

It is essential to note that these are not the only possible interactions. Always inform your healthcare provider of all medications, supplements, and substances you are using. They will be able to evaluate the potential interactions and determine whether or not you can safely take Viagra. If necessary, your healthcare provider may modify your medication regimen, suggest an alternative treatment, or provide guidelines to reduce the risk of potential drug interactions.

Never initiate, discontinue, or alter the dosage of any medication without the supervision of a qualified healthcare professional. For a safe and effective treatment experience with Viagra or any other medication, it is vital to maintain open communication with your healthcare provider.

Addressing common concerns and misconceptions

Individuals can make more informed decisions about the use of Viagra (sildenafil citrate) to treat erectile dysfunction if they are informed about prevalent concerns and misconceptions about the drug. Here are a few of the most common misconceptions and concerns, along with the correct information to clarify them:

Concern: Viagra Increases Sexual Desire • Misconception: Some people believe Viagra is a "libido booster" that increases sexual desire.

Viagra is not an aphrodisiac and has no effect on sexual desire or arousal. It functions by increasing blood flow to the penis, thereby assisting in the attainment and maintenance of an erection in response to sexual stimulation.

Concern: Viagra Causes Unintentional Erections

• Misconception: It is commonly believed that Viagra induces spontaneous erections in the absence of sexual stimulation.

Viagra enhances the natural response of the organism to sexual stimulation. It does not cause spontaneous erections; sexual arousal is still required for the procedure to begin.

Concern: Viagra Is Dependent

• Misconception: Some individuals believe that using Viagra can contribute to addiction or dependency.

• Viagra is not addictive, as a fact. It is a medication prescribed for intermittent treatment of erectile dysfunction. It does not establish a habit.

4. Fear: Viagra Works Instantaneously
• Misconception: Some individuals expect Viagra to begin working immediately after administration.

• While Viagra's onset of action can be comparatively quick, it typically takes between 30 minutes and an hour to take effect. Food consumption and an individual's reaction time can affect its effectiveness.

Concern: Young Men Do Not Need Viagra • Misconception: Erectile dysfunction is commonly associated with aging, leading some younger men to believe they do not require Viagra.

• Erectile dysfunction can affect men of all ages, and its fundamental causes can vary. Viagra can benefit younger men with erectile dysfunction caused by psychological factors, lifestyle choices, or medical conditions.

Concern: Viagra Treats the Root Causes of ED

• Misconception: Some believe Viagra treats the root causes of erectile dysfunction.

Viagra alleviates the symptoms of erectile dysfunction by increasing blood flow to the penile. Although it can be effective, it does not address the underlying causes of erectile dysfunction, which may include hormonal imbalances or cardiovascular problems.

7. Fear: Viagra Is Reserved for Extreme ED Cases

• Misconception: It is a common misconception that Viagra is only appropriate for men with acute erectile dysfunction.

Viagra can be prescribed for mild to severe cases of erectile dysfunction.

Professionals in the medical field evaluate individual requirements and may recommend Viagra based on a variety of factors.

8. Fear: Viagra Guarantees Immediate Success • Misconception: Some individuals anticipate immediate success with Viagra and may become disheartened if the results are not instantaneous.

Viagra's efficacy differs from individual to individual. Achieving the desired result may require multiple attempts or dosage adjustments.

9. Fear: Viagra Is a Permanent Fix • Myth: Some individuals believe that a single use of Viagra will perpetually resolve their erectile dysfunction.

Viagra is a temporary treatment for erectile dysfunction symptoms. It is not a permanent remedy. It is necessary to address the underlying causes, and treatment plans may include lifestyle modifications or other interventions.

Accurately addressing these concerns and misconceptions about Viagra's effects and its position in the treatment of erectile dysfunction enables individuals to have realistic expectations regarding the drug's efficacy. For a comprehensive approach to managing ED and making informed treatment decisions, open communication with healthcare professionals is essential.

CHAPTER SIX

Testimonials from individuals who have experienced positive effects

Certainly, the following are fictitious testimonials from men who have experienced positive results from using Viagra (sildenafil citrate) to treat erectile dysfunction:

1. John, 52: "Viagra has genuinely transformed my life. I decided to test it after years of struggling with erectile dysfunction. The results were astounding. Not only did I regain the ability to attain and maintain an erection, but my confidence and self-esteem also increased substantially. My relationship with my companion has never been stronger since this

realization. Viagra has breathed fresh vitality into me."

Sarah, age 45: "I was initially cautious about using Viagra, but my physician assured me that it was a safe and effective option. I am so happy I followed their advice. Viagra has significantly altered my relationship with my spouse. Our closeness and connection have vastly improved. It's also about the emotional closeness that accompanies the physical proximity. I regret not having attempted it sooner!"

David, 37: "Having erectile dysfunction as a relatively young male was exasperating and humiliating. I believed it was something that only affected elderly men. However, my physician explained that ED can affect men of any age. He suggested Viagra, and I can honestly say it has changed the game. I have regained my former confidence, vitality, and commitment to my relationship. Viagra restored the intimacy I believed I had lost."

4. Emily, age 31: "My companion and I observed a change in our intimate life after the birth of our first child. It was affecting our relationship, and I felt bad that I was unable to satisfy his needs. We chose to investigate our options and learned about Viagra. It was an enlightenment. It not only helped us reestablish our physical connection, but it also reignited our emotional connection. Due to Viagra, our relationship is stronger than ever."

5. Mike, 58: "When I reached my late 50s, I accepted that my sexual life would never be the same. Viagra, however, proven me incorrect. For my bedroom activities, it's like a fountain of vitality. My partner and I are experiencing an unprecedented level of intimacy. It has brought us closer together, rekindled our passion, and provided us with a renewed sense of vitality."

Please note that these testimonials are fictitious and are intended to illustrate the positive experiences that some users of Viagra may have. Before using any medication for erectile dysfunction, it is essential to consult a healthcare professional because individual experiences can vary.

Addressing misconceptions and stigma surrounding Viagra use

In order to promote open and enlightened discussions about erectile dysfunction (ED) and its treatment, it is crucial to dispel common myths and stigmas surrounding Viagra use. Here are some strategies for dispelling misconceptions and reducing stigma:

• Providing accurate information about Viagra, its mechanism of action, benefits, and limitations can help dispel falsehoods and misunderstandings.

• Inform the public that Viagra is a treatment for the physical symptoms of erectile dysfunction and does not effect desire or arousal.

Normalizing Erectile Dysfunction as a Medical Condition: • Stress that ED is a medical condition, similar to other health issues, that can affect men of any age.

• Emphasize that seeking treatment for erectile dysfunction is comparable to seeking treatment for any other medical condition.

• Encourage individuals to have open and honest conversations about ED with their companions, healthcare providers, and support networks.

• Normalize conversations about sexual health, making it simpler for individuals to seek advice and assistance.

Sharing Personal Experiences: • Sharing the personal experiences of those who have benefited from Viagra or other ED treatments can help reduce the stigma associated with erectile dysfunction.

• Personal narratives can shed light on the emotional and relational effects of ED and the positive effects of treatment on individuals' lives.

• Dispel the fallacy that ED is exclusively an age-related issue. Explain that erectile dysfunction can be caused by a variety of factors, including medical conditions, lifestyle, stress, and psychological issues.

6. Emphasizing Individuality: • Understand that each person's response to Viagra may differ. Others may experience significantly different outcomes, while some may experience significant improvement.

7. Promoting Holistic Health: •
Emphasize that managing ED
frequently requires a holistic approach,
including lifestyle modifications,
treatment of underlying health
conditions, and emotional support.

• Encourage individuals to seek
guidance from healthcare professionals
who can provide accurate information,
address concerns, and provide
individualized treatment plans.

• Challenge preconceived notions about
masculinity and sexual performance
that contribute to stigma.

• Encourage an inclusive conception of
relationships, intimacy, and self-worth.

• Promote awareness campaigns that
emphasize the significance of sexual
health, de-stigmatize ED, and

encourage individuals to seek assistance without embarrassment.

Reducing the stigma and misconceptions surrounding Viagra use and erectile dysfunction is a group effort involving healthcare professionals, educators, advocates, and individuals. By fostering frank conversations, disseminating accurate information, and promoting a compassionate and understanding attitude, we can create a more supportive environment for those coping with erectile dysfunction and seeking effective treatments such as Viagra.

About the Author

Dr. Billy Rich is a distinguished figure in the field of urology and sexual health, with a passion for helping individuals reclaim their vitality and confidence. With years of experience as a practicing urologist, Dr. Rich has dedicated his career to addressing the unique challenges that impact intimate relationships.

A graduate of the prestigious University of California, San Francisco, Dr. Rich has cultivated a deep understanding of the physical and psychological aspects of sexual health. His expertise has guided countless patients toward holistic solutions, emphasizing the importance of open communication, informed choices, and personalized care.

Dr. Rich's commitment to spreading awareness and knowledge led him to pen "Viagra Med." This comprehensive guide is a culmination of his clinical insights, scientific expertise, and a genuine desire to empower individuals and couples to overcome erectile dysfunction (ED) and embrace a renewed sense of intimacy.

As an author, Dr. Rich simplifies complex medical concepts, making them accessible to readers seeking answers and solutions. His approach is not just clinical; it's compassionate. "Viagra Med" reflects Dr. Rich's dedication to enhancing lives, rekindling relationships, and fostering a sense of self-assuredness that goes beyond the pages.

With "Viagra Med," Dr. Billy Rich invites you to embark on a journey of rediscovery and transformation. Let his expertise be your guide as you navigate the path to renewed vitality and intimate connection.

Printed in Great Britain
by Amazon

28016388R00046